Intermittent Fasting For Women Of Over 50

The Ultimate 101 Guide to Mastering Healthy Weight Loss as an Aging Woman - Support your Hormones and Detox Your Body with this 16/8 Plan and Selected Recipes

Amanda Harper

Table of Contents

INTRODUCTION 4

CHAPTER I Intermittent Fasting for Women Over 50 7

CHAPTER II 14

Types Of Intermittent Fasting 14

CHAPTER III 20

Pros and Cons of Intermittent Fasting 20

CHAPTER IV 25

What Foods Are Best to Eat on an Intermittent Fasting Diet? 25

CHAPTER V 29

Intermittent Fasting For Weight Loss Tips 29

CHAPTER VI 34

Intermittent Fasting Recipes 34
    Keto Buffalo Wing Chicken Salad 34
    Low Carb Taco Salad 36
    Low-Carb Cheese & Bacon Stuffed Meat Pies 38
    Healthy scrambled eggs 40
    Moroccan baked eggs 42
    Low-Carb Butter Braised Cabbage with Crispy Ham 44
    Vegetables With Red Pepper Rouille 45
    Garlic Mushroom Frittata 47
    Stir-Fried Pork With Ginger And Soy Sauce 49
    Salmon BLTs 51
    Italian style meatballs with courgette 'tagliatelle' 53
    Chilli And Coriander Fish Parcel 55
    Extra-Lean Burger And Salad 57
    Red mullet with baked tomatoes 59
    Chicken And Vegetable Balti 61

Poached Eggs With Bacon And Tomatoes 63
Peppered Beef With Salad Leaves 64
Lamb And Flageolet Bean Stew 66
Chermoula Tofu And Roasted Vegetables 68
Hearty Vegetable Soup 70
Caponata Ratatouille 72
Italian Omelet 74
Keto Crispy Ginger Mackerel Lunch Bowl 76
Smoked Salmon, Avocado & Egg Lunch Bowl 78
Speedy Low-Carb Tuna Lunch Bowl 81
Low-Carb Veggie Full English Breakfast Bowl 83
Low-Carb Chocolate Coconut Smoothie 85
Healthy Salmon & Tabbouleh Low-Carb Bowl 87
Bacon, Egg & Asparagus Keto Bowl 90
Easy Pork Chops With Asparagus and Hollandaise 93
Low-Carb All Day Mexican Bowl 95
Anti Keto Flu Nourish Bowl 97
Keto Portobello Mushroom Mini Pizzas 99
Sugar-Free Lemon Granita 101

CONCLUSION 104

INTRODUCTION

Intermittent fasting has become quietly popular in circles where people are striving to come up with ways to reduce caloric intake without harming their workout goals and still allow them to lose weight while strength training.

Intermittent fasting in a nutshell is the practice of short-term fasts that are 24 hours in length and done once or twice per week. There are variations on that theme, but in general, that is the norm. This is done not so much to "cleanse the system" as many would have you believe, though it will to a certain degree. It's merely a simple and fast way of decreasing caloric intake so you can achieve your weight loss goals without starvation plans or other fad diets. You don't have to be overly concerned about the types of food you consume while you're not fasting, although it should be noted that fasting once or twice per week won't really help you reach your goals if you spend the other five or six days stuffing yourself with all manner of junk. A bit more care and consciousness is required.

By allowing a sense of freedom in your food choices, it relieves a great deal of the anxiety present when it comes to most diets. Many times we feel totally constrained and restricted. However, this approach leaves us being able to not only choose what we'd like to consume, but also brings balance and sanity back into our diets. Intermittent fasting as a lifestyle will bring about changes that will last a lifetime. Start by taking it slow at first, and really learn to listen to what your body is trying to tell you as you go through your first few weeks of this. If you find yourself feeling lethargic or underfed, change it up a bit. Your body will tell you what it needs. (And that usually isn't a monster double cheeseburger!) Many times, especially at first, your body will be going through some withdrawals, and it's important to learn how to differentiate the signals. Also, you need to factor in what effect any workout routines you may be involved in will have on your intermittent fasting plans.

The most important thing to remember about intermittent fasting is that it is not merely a diet plan, but a lifestyle, worthy of consideration along those lines. In order to get the best results possible from this type of plan, you need to befriend it. Your fasting should be something that you look forward to, as you most certainly will after you start reaping some of the benefits of this intermittent fasting lifestyle. Making this type of plan fits into your life is key to making a lifetime of good eating and healthy living possible. There are a lot of inherent freedoms built into a diet plan like this, and while that can backfire on you if you're not careful, it can also enable lasting success.

CHAPTER I

Intermittent Fasting for Women Over 50

The pattern of eating called "Intermittent Fasting" usually means one fasts for a period of time and eats for a period of time. Many choose a 24-hour cycle of fasting, then eat healthy the next day, and continue this process as a lifestyle change. Intermittent fasting has become a popular and best way for Women of over 50 to use the body's natural fat-burning ability to lose fat in a short period of time.

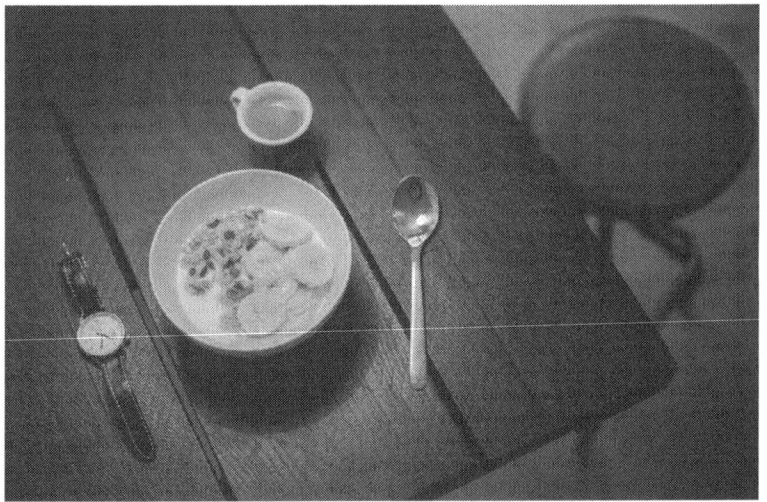

Research has been done on animals to find the benefits of this type of fasting, and you will be happy to know it really can be beneficial to your health!

Intermittent fasting can add 40%-56% more years to your life! That in itself is reason enough to do it. However, other benefits include body weight reduction and fat oxidation.

When you fast, your body is forced to scavenge for fuel, thus removing aged and damaged cells in the process. This sort of fast cleanses the body of undesirable and unwanted things and helps the weight loss and benefits of the good food choices to be increased and more beneficial to your body.

Rats have been shown to have long-term and improved survival after heart failure when placed on an IF eating plan, too. Researchers are also saying that it might help age related deficits in cognitive function, too, so that tells me that it might help ward off Alzheimer's Disease and other types of Dementia!

Your risk of heart disease and other heart ailments may also be decreased when you start a healthy and intermittent fasting regimen. Your risk for other chronic illnesses and diseases will also most likely be reduced.

A healthier you can begin with intermittent fasting and healthy food choices! Keep carbs to 50-100 grams per day. Many women eat between 1200-1500 calories per day, and when limiting their carbs, they are still losing weight. Men can handle up to 2000 calories per day. Of course, less is best, and you need to determine caloric intake based on your activities such as working hard and exercising.

Drink lots of fluids, especially water and exercise in the evenings if possible. This will help with those late-night cravings.

Once you start eating and drinking healthier, your body won't crave as much (if any) junk food, so making healthy food choices will simply get easier and easier as you progress in the intermittent fasting routine.

Alternate Day Fasting or ADF means alternating days of eating and not eating any food, but there is also an intermittent fasting called Modified Fasting, where you consume about 20% of your normal calories one day and then eat normally (but healthy) the next day. This is often more attainable for people because they feel less deprived when they are able to at least eat something daily, and it still has most of the benefits of the ADF regimen.

What Is Intermittent Fasting?

It has different meanings to different people. From a simple overnight fast of 12 hours that we would all benefit from to not eating between meals (forgo the eat 6 times a day and every 2-3 hours mandate), to going days without anything but juice or water, there's a wide range to choose from.

Lately though, the most popular forms getting attention are fasting for 16-18 hours at a time. For most, that's not eating until noon. Since going to bed hungry is counter to one of the objectives of IF, which is to increase Growth Hormone, skipping dinner is less appealing. Tossing and turning due to hunger will decrease the production of GH, the greatest of which is done during deep sleep phases.

That flies in the face of breakfast being the most important meal of the day. And really goes counter to studies suggesting starting the day with the highest ingestion of protein, which will enhance choices all day if not fat metabolism.

For women over 50 who are regularly active, but still struggles with fat loss, intermittent fasting can help to increase fat loss without having to ramp up a workout regime or drastically alter a diet plan.

Is It Right For You?

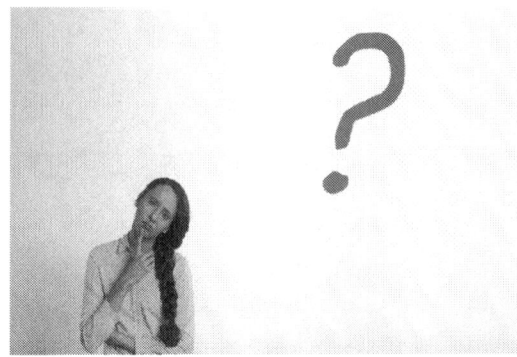

Consider times you've gone without food for long periods. If you're currently flirting with intermittent fasting (whether consciously or your dieting mentality has crept into your food control), ask the following:

- Do you feel weaker or have less endurance?
- Have you noticed the same workouts feel more difficult?
- Is your quality of sleep suffering?
- Do you feel any lack of concentration or focus?
- Do you feel more anxious, depressed, or lack memory?
- Are you noticeably distracted by hunger?

How Intermittent Fasting Works

Intermittent fasting simply means you go a period without eating, usually between 12 to 48 hours. This is known as your fasting window, during which time you only consume liquids, such as water, herbal tea or broth.

Some experts recommend drinking low-calorie green vegetable juices and taking supplements, while fasting to help keep vitamin and mineral intake consistent. There are others though, who believe only water should be consumed. Like many topics in the health realm, the rules around intermittent fasting are subjective, depending on who you ask.

If you fast for less than 24 hours, you'll also have an eating window. This is the time allotted for meals before you begin your fast. For most people practicing intermittent fasting, their eating window is between six to 12 hours: the most common fasting times are 12, 14, 16, and 18 hours.

For example, if you were to do a 12-hour fast, your eating window would be 12 hours. You could start your eating window at 7AM and end at 7PM. You would break the fast the next day at 7AM.

Although some of the intermittent fasting Instructions online seem more intense than others (some can last upwards of 48 hours), the beauty of intermittent fasting is that you get to choose and experiment with how long you fast. This not only allows you to determine how intermittent fasting can fit in within your lifestyle, but to discover the fasting sweet spot that helps you feel best physically.

CHAPTER II

Types Of Intermittent Fasting

Intermittent fasting comes in various forms and each may have a specific set of unique benefits. Each form of intermittent fasting has variations in the fasting-to-eating ratio. The benefits and effectiveness of these different protocols may differ on an individual basis and it is important to determine which one is best for you. Factors that may influence which one to choose include health goals, daily schedule/routine, and current health status. The most common types of IF are alternate day fasting, time-restricted feeding, and modified fasting.

Alternate Day Fasting

This approach involves alternating between days of absolutely no calories, from food or beverage, with days of free feeding and eating whatever you want.

This plan has been shown to help with weight loss, improve blood cholesterol and triglyceride (fat) levels, and improve markers for inflammation in the blood.

The main downfall with this form of intermittent fasting is that it is the most difficult to stick with because of the reported hunger during fasting days.

The Warrior Diet

The Warrior Diet is a relatively extreme form of intermittent fasting.

The Warrior Diet involves eating very little, usually just a few servings of raw fruit and vegetables, during a 20-hour fasting window, then eating one large meal at night. The eating window is usually only around 4 hours.

This form of fasting may be best for people who have tried other forms of intermittent fasting already.

Supporters of the Warrior Diet claim that humans are natural nocturnal eaters and that eating at night allows the body to gain nutrients in line with its circadian rhythms.

During the 4-hour eating phase, people should make sure that they consume plenty of vegetables, proteins, and healthy fats. They should also include some carbohydrates.

Although it is possible to eat some foods during the fasting period, it can be challenging to stick to the strict guidelines on when and what to eat in the long term. Also, some people struggle with eating such a large meal so close to bedtime.

Meal skipping

This flexible approach to intermittent fasting may be good for beginners. It involves occasionally skipping meals.

People can decide which meals to skip according to their level of hunger or time restraints. However, it is important to eat healthful foods at each meal.

Meal skipping is likely to be most successful when individuals monitor and respond to their body's hunger signals. Essentially, people using this style of intermittent fasting will eat when they are hungry and skip meals when they are not.

Modified Fasting - 5:2 Diet

Modified fasting is a protocol with programmed fasting days, but the fasting days do allow for some food intake. Generally, 20-25% of normal calories are allowed to be consumed on fasting days; so if you normally consume 2000 calories on regular eating days, you would be allowed 400-500 calories on fasting days. The 5:2 part of this diet refers to the ratio of non-fasting to fasting days. So on this regimen, you would normally eat for 5 consecutive days, then fast or restrict calories to 20-25% for 2 consecutive days.

This protocol is great for weight loss, body composition, and may also benefit the regulation of blood sugar, lipids, and inflammation. Studies have shown the 5:2 protocol to be effective for weight loss, improve/lower inflammation markers in the blood (3), and show signs trending improvements in insulin resistance. In animal studies, this modified fasting 5:2 diet resulted in decreased fat, decreased hunger hormones (leptin), and increased levels of a protein responsible for improvements in fat burning and blood sugar regulation (adiponectin).

The modified 5:2 fasting protocol is easy to follow and has a small number of negative side effects, which includes hunger, low energy, and some irritability when beginning the program. Contrary to this, however, studies have also noted improvements such as reduced tension, less anger, less fatigue, improvements in self confidence, and a more positive mood.

A Weekly 24-Hour Fast

On a 24-hour diet, a person can have teas and calorie-free drinks.

Fasting completely for 1 or 2 days a week, known as the Eat-Stop-Eat diet, involves eating no food for 24 hours at a time. Many people fast from breakfast to breakfast or lunch to lunch.

People on this diet plan can have water, tea, and other calorie-free drinks during the fasting period.

People should return to normal eating patterns on the non-fasting days. Eating in this manner reduces a person's total calorie intake but does not limit the specific foods that the individual consumes.

A 24-hour fast can be challenging, and it may cause fatigue, headaches, or irritability. Many people find that these effects become less extreme over time as the body adjusts to this new pattern of eating.

People may benefit from trying a 12-hour or 16-hour fast before transitioning to the 24-hour fast.

Time-Restricted Feeding

If you know anyone that has said they are doing intermittent fasting, odds are it is in the form of time-restricted feeding. This is a type of intermittent fasting that is used daily. It involves only consuming calories during a small portion of the day and fasting for the remainder. Daily fasting intervals in time-restricted feeding may range from 12-20 hours, with the most common instruction being 16/8 (fasting for 16 hours, consuming calories for 8). For this protocol, the time of day is not important as long as you are fasting for a consecutive period of time and only eating in your allowed time period. For example, on a 16/8 time-restricted feeding program one person may eat their first meal at 7AM and last meal at 3PM (fast from 3PM-7AM), while another person may eat their first meal at 1PM and last meal at 9PM (fast from 9PM-1PM). This protocol is meant to be performed every day over long periods of time and is very flexible as long as you are staying within the fasting/eating window(s).

Time-Restricted feeding is one of the easiest to follow instructions of intermittent fasting. Using this, along with your daily work and sleep schedule may help achieve optimal metabolic function. Time-restricted feeding is a great program to follow for weight loss and body composition improvements as well as some other Prep/Cook Time: health benefits. The few human trials that were conducted, noted significant reductions in weight, reductions in fasting blood glucose, and improvements in cholesterol with no changes in perceived tension, depression, anger, fatigue, or confusion. Some other preliminary results from animal studies showed time restricted feeding to protect against obesity, high insulin levels, fatty liver disease, and inflammation.

The easy application and promising results of time-restricted feeding could possibly make it an excellent option for weight loss and chronic disease prevention/management. When implementing this protocol, it may be good to begin with a lower fasting-to-eating ratio like 12/12 hours and eventually work your way up to 16/8 hours.

CHAPTER III

Pros and Cons of Intermittent Fasting

If you are thinking about starting an intermittent fasting protocol for weight loss, it can be one of the best decisions you make.

That being said, there are many pros and cons to intermittent fasting. It's best to take some time and go through in-depth thought and research before making a commitment.

Pros

Intermittent Fasting and Cancer in Older Women

Fasting for different lengths of time also helped middle age women reduce their risk of serious diseases with much of the research focused on the positive effects fasting has on cancer.

The study stated that fasting seems to inhibit some of the pathways that lead to cancer and can also slow the growth of tumors.

You will have more energy.

Since you will not eat as much, there will be less wavering of blood sugar levels. This means that real energy will be more consistent. Plus, you lessen the risk of getting diabetes. You can also exercise while you are on fast which will actually boost your body's potential to burn more fats. A growth hormone is increased when you fast, which helps to burn calories.

IF Improves Muscle and Joint Health

The researchers also found that fasting improved muscle and joint health, so things like arthritic symptoms and low back pain were not as pronounced.

Intermittent Fasting for Women Over 50 Joint Health

They reviewed a few studies conducted and it showed that periods of fasting affected the way your body produces the hormones that affect bone minerals like calcium and phosphate. Therefore, it had some indication linking periods of fasting to improved bone health.

You burn more fat which means weight loss.

Since you eat less and are taking in fewer calories, your body will turn into body fat to burn for energy. This happens instead of your body taking the energy from the food that is otherwise eaten on a regular basis if you are not on Intermittent Fasting. This also means that your body will show more of fit, lean, muscle mass. On a side note, if you are fasting for about 16 hours, your body is already consuming body fat.

You keep yourself full.

Some people think that fasting or dieting for that matter is equal to starvation. However, when Intermittent Fasting is done, Ghrelin, which is a hormone that signals hunger, adjusts to the new way of eating of the body and this is why you will not feel hungry.

You will have better focus and improved concentration.

When fasting, catecholamines, which is another hormone of the body, is produced more. Therefore, the end result is that you will be more focused on what you are doing.

Intermittent Fasting and Depression

The review study also took into consideration mental health aspects and highlighted many studies showing that women who practice different fasting techniques saw improvement in their moods, self-esteem and had a decrease in anxiety and depression.

Cons

No Focus on Nutritious Eating

The cornerstone of most intermittent fasting programs is timing, rather than food choice. Therefore no foods (including those that lack good nutrition) are avoided and foods that provide good nutrition are not promoted. For this reason, those following the diet don't necessarily learn to eat a healthy diet.

If you are following a short-term intermittent fasting program for weight loss or to gain a medical benefit, it is not likely that you will learn basic healthy eating and cooking skills, including how to cook with healthy oils, how to eat more vegetables, and how to choose whole grains over refined grains.

Severe Hunger

Not surprisingly, it is common for those in the fasting stage of an IF eating plan to experience severe hunger. This hunger may become more extreme when they are around others who are consuming typical meals and snacks.

Medications

Many people who take medications find that taking their prescription with food helps to relieve certain side effects. In fact, some medications specifically carry the recommendation that they should be taken with food. Therefore, taking medications during fasting may be a challenge.

May Promote Overeating

During the "feasting" stage of many intermittent fasting protocols, meal size and meal frequency are not restricted. Instead, consumers enjoy an ad libitum diet. Unfortunately, this may promote overeating in some people. For example, if you feel deprived after a day of complete fasting, you may feel inclined to overeat (or eat the wrong foods) on days when "feasting" is allowed.

Reduced Physical Activity

One notable side effect of intermittent fasting may be the reduction of physical activity. Most intermittent fasting programs do not include a recommendation for physical activity. Not surprisingly, those who follow the programs may experience enough fatigue that they fail to meet daily step goals and may even change their regular exercise routines.

Ongoing research is underway to see how intermittent fasting may affect physical activity patterns.

CHAPTER IV

What Foods Are Best to Eat on an Intermittent Fasting Diet?

There are no specifications or restrictions about what type or how much food to eat while following intermittent fasting," says Lauren Harris-Pincus, MS, RDN, author of The Protein-Packed Breakfast Club.

Beans and Legumes

Your favorite addition to chili may be your best friend on the IF lifestyle. Food, specifically carbs, supplies energy for activity. While we're not telling you to carbo-load, it definitely would not hurt to throw some low-calorie carbs, like beans and legumes, into your eating plan. Plus, foods like chickpeas, black beans, peas, and lentils have been shown to decrease body weight, even without calorie restriction.

Berries

Your favorite smoothie addition is ripe with vital nutrients. Strawberries are a great source of immune-boosting vitamin C, with more than 100 percent of the daily value in one cup. And that's not even the best part—a recent study found that people who consumed a diet rich in flavonoids, like those in blueberries and strawberries, had smaller increases in BMI over a 14-year period than those who did not eat berries.

Eggs

One large egg has six grams of protein and cooks in minutes. Getting as much protein as possible is important for keeping full and building muscle. One study found that men who ate an egg for breakfast instead of a bagel were less hungry and ate less throughout the day. In other words, when you're looking for something to do during your fasting period, why not hard-boil some eggs?

Probiotics

You know what the little critters in your gut like the most? Consistency and diversity. That means they aren't happy when they're hungry and when your gut isn't happy, you may experience some irritating side effects, like constipation. To counteract this unpleasantness, add probiotic-rich foods, like kefir, kombucha or kraut, to your diet. The Farmhouse Culture Gut Shots are perfect for any 500-calorie days, since each 1.5-ounce shot is brimming with live probiotics (10 billion CFUs) for just 10 calories.

Nuts

They may be higher in calories than many other snacks, but nuts contain something that most junk food doesn't—good fat. Research suggests that polyunsaturated fat in walnuts can actually alter the physiological markers for hunger and satiety.

And if you're worried about calories, don't be! A 2012 study found that a one-ounce serving of almonds (about 23 nuts) has 20 percent fewer calories than listed on the label. Basically, the chewing process does not completely break down the almond cell walls, leaving a portion of the nut intact and unabsorbed during digestion.

Whole Grains

Being on a diet and eating carbs seem like they belong in two different buckets, but not always! Whole grains are rich in fiber and protein, so eating a little goes a long way in keeping you full. Plus, a new study suggests that eating whole grains instead of refined grains may actually rev up your metabolism. So, go ahead and eat your whole grains and venture out of your comfort zone to try farro, bulgur, spelt, kamut, amaranth, millet, sorghum, or freekeh.

Cruciferous Veggies

Foods like broccoli, Brussels sprouts, and cauliflower are all full of the f-word—fiber. When you're eating erratically, it's crucial to eat fiber-rich foods that will keep you regular and prevent constipation. Fiber also has the ability to make you feel full, which is something you may want if you can't eat again for 16 hours. Woof.

Potatoes

Not all white foods are bad. Case in point: Studies found potatoes to be one of the most satiating foods around. Another study found that eating potatoes as part of a healthy diet could help with weight loss. Sorry, French fries and potato chips don't count.

CHAPTER V

Intermittent Fasting For Weight Loss Tips

Here are some tips to help you understand the concept accurately and implement it more effectively.

Eat Enough Protein

Many people start fasting as a way to try to lose weight.

However, being in a calorie deficit can cause you to lose muscle in addition to fat.

One way to minimize your muscle loss while fasting is to ensure you are eating enough protein on the days you eat.

Additionally, if you are eating small amounts on fast days, including some protein, it could offer other benefits, including managing your hunger.

Some studies suggest that consuming around 30% of a meal's calories from protein can significantly reduce your appetite.

Therefore, eating some protein on fast days could help offset some of the fasting's side effects.

Going extreme isn't always better

Popular IF advice online says to abstain for 16 to 24 hours between feeding periods on a regular basis. However, a feeding window of 12 hours per day is ideal for optimal health.

While the diet psychology of IF clearly appeals to some people, even done short term, conventional IF advice may come with health risks.

If you eat only for four to six hours a day, "then you start to see gallstone formation [and] increase the chance that you're [going to] need your gallbladder removed."

Studies show that elongated periods between eating increases the risk of gallstone formation in women, regardless of weight.

While research hasn't found the exact connection, studies by Trusted Source, indicatesthat people who skip breakfast tend to have much higher rates of cancer, cardiovascular disease, and death.

Extreme, limited feeding windows and alternate-day fasting can also cause problems with cardiovascular disease, whereas 12-hour TRF was shown in a study on flies to decrease age-related cardiac decline. Trusted Source.

On the other end of the spectrum, Longo notes that "if you eat 15 hours a day or more, that starts to be associated with metabolic problems, sleep disorders, etc."

Eat for 12 hours, then refrain for the next 12. Stick as closely to this daily feeding schedule as possible to minimize adverse health effects.

Consider Supplements

If you fast regularly, you may miss out on essential nutrients.

This is because regularly eating fewer calories makes it harder to meet your nutritional needs.

In fact, people following weight loss diets are more likely to be deficient in a number of essential nutrients like iron, calcium and vitamin B12.

As such, those who fast regularly should consider taking a multivitamin for peace of mind and to help prevent deficiencies.

Basically, it's always best to get your nutrients from whole foods.

Stop Fasting If You Feel Unwell

During a fast, you may feel a little tired, hungry and irritable — but you should never feel unwell.

To keep yourself safe, especially if you are new to fasting, consider limiting your fast periods to 24 hours or fewer and keeping a snack on hand in case you start to feel faint or ill.

If you do become ill or are concerned about your health, make sure you stop fasting straight away.

Some signs that you should stop your fast and seek medical help include tiredness or weakness that prevents you from carrying out daily tasks, as well as unexpected feelings of sickness and discomfort.

Eat Plenty of Whole Foods on Non-Fasting Days

Most people who fast are trying to improve their health.

Even though fasting involves abstaining from food, it's still important to maintain a healthy lifestyle on days when you are not fasting.

Healthy diets based on whole foods are linked to a wide range of health benefits, including a reduced risk of cancer, heart disease, and other chronic illnesses.

You can make sure your diet remains healthy by choosing whole foods like meat, fish, eggs, vegetables, fruits, and legumes when you eat.

Keep Exercise Mild

Some people find that they are able to maintain their regular exercise regimen while fasting (5Trusted Source).

However, if you're new to fasting, it's best to keep any exercise to a low intensity — especially at first — so you can see how you manage.

Low-intensity exercises could include walking, mild yoga, gentle stretching, and housework.

Most importantly, listen to your body and rest if you struggle to exercise while fasting.

CHAPTER VI

Intermittent Fasting Recipes

Here are delicious selected recipes for your meals.

Keto Buffalo Wing Chicken Salad

Recipe type: Entree
Prep time: 10 mins
Cook time: 10 mins
Total time: 20 mins
Serves: 2 servings

Ingredients

- 2 heads Romaine Lettuce, chopped
- ½ cup Provel Cheese, shredded
- 3 slices of bacon, chopped and cooked
- ¼ cup Pico de Gallo
- 8oz Chicken Breast
- ½ cup Wing Sauce (only about ¼ cup ends up in the salad)
- Salt & Pepper, to taste
- ¼ cup Buttermilk Ranch Dressing

Instructions

- Grill the chicken breast in a skillet over medium-high heat. Season with salt and pepper.
- Sear each side for 3-4 minutes until nicely browned, then flip to brown the other side. Lower the heat down to medium, and cook for an additional 8 minutes (depending on how thick the chicken breast is) until cooked through.

- Let the grilled chicken breast rest for 5 minutes on a cutting board, then slice into strips and toss in the wing sauce.
- In the hot skillet, chop the raw bacon (or cut with kitchen shears: my favorite instruction) and cook until browned. Drain and set aside.
- While the chicken cooks and/or rests, assemble the salad.
- Chop the romaine lettuce, then place into a bowl with the cheese, pico de gallo, and the Buttermilk Ranch. Toss to combine.
- Place the tossed salad in a large serving bowl.
- Top the salad with the chopped & cooked bacon and grilled buffalo chicken. Serve immediately.

Low Carb Taco Salad

A healthy taco salad, using wholesome ingredients, is naturally low in carbs, easy to prepare, and absolutely delicious! Use lean ground beef or turkey.

Prep Time: 15 minutes
Cook Time: 10 minutes
Total Time: 25 minutes
Servings: 4
Calories: 530

Ingredients

- 1 pound lean ground beef
- 2 whole Romaine hearts (340 grams), chopped
- 1 whole avocado, cubed
- 4 ounce cheddar cheese, cubed
- 3 ounces grape tomatoes, halved
- 2 tbsp sliced red onion (½ ounce)
- 1 tsp ground cumin (or 2 tbsp of Homemade Taco Seasoning)
- salt and pepper to taste

Mexican Viniagrette

- ½ batch Cilantro Lime Vinaigrette (sub sugar-free sweetener to taste, for the honey)

Optional Ingredients:

- salsa
- sour cream

Instructions

- Make vinaigrette per instructions. Chop and prepare vegetables and cheese.

- Place the ground beef in a cold pan over medium heat. Work the ground beef in the pan to break up into tiny crumbles, about 7 minutes. Add the cumin and salt and pepper to taste. Alternately, use 2 tbsp of my homemade taco seasoning. Let cool slightly.
- Place all of the ingredients into a large bowl and toss with the dressing. Top with a dollop of sour cream and salsa if desired (don't forget to count the carbs). Serves 4.

Nutrition Info

Calories: 530
Calories from Fat 378
Fat: 42g 65%
Sodium: 408mg 18%
Carbohydrates: 9g 3%
Fiber: 5g 21%
Protein: 32g 64%

Low-Carb Cheese & Bacon Stuffed Meat Pies

Prep/Cook Time: 50 min
Servings: 4

Ingredients

Filling:

- 500 g ground beef (1.1 lb)
- 4 large slices bacon, chopped (120 g/ 4.2 oz)
- 1 small brown onion, chopped (g/ oz)
- 1 tbsp coconut aminos (15 ml)
- 2 tbsp tomato sauce/passata (30 ml)
- 1 cup beef stock or bone broth (240 ml/ 8 fl oz)
- ½ tsp xanthan gum

Pie crust:

- 2 ¼ cups shredded mozzarella cheese (250g/8.8oz)
- 1 cup 2 tbsp shredded edam cheese (125g/4.4oz)
- 1/3 cup 1 tbsp full-fat cream cheese (100g/3.5oz)
- 1 ½ cups almond flour (150g/5.3oz)
- 2 large eggs
- 1 tsp onion powder
- 6 small chunks of sharp cheddar (66g/2.3oz)

Instructions

- Cut the bacon into small strips and dice the onion.
- Add to a skillet, along with the ground beef. Cook until just browned.

- Add coconut aminos, passata, beef stock, and xanthan gum and stir well to combine. Bring to boil then reduce the heat and simmer for 30 minutes.
- Remove from the heat and let cool. Once mixture is cool, heat oven to 200 °C/ 390 °F (fan assisted).
- Prepare the pie crust. Place the cheeses and cream cheese into a large bowl and microwave for 1 minute. Remove and stir, then return for another 30 seconds. Repeat this once more. Add the almond meal, onion powder and eggs and mix well until you have a soft dough.
- Divide into four parts and sit one portion aside. Cut each of the remaining three portions in half and then flatten them out into large circles (you will have a total of six circles).
- Spray a six-hole oversized muffin pan and press the dough into each cup, making sure to leave overhang at the top as the dough will shrink while cooking. Bake for 10 minutes.
- Remove and spoon some filling into each cup. Press a chunk of cheddar into the centre.
- Then top with the remaining filling.
- Divide the reserved dough into six and flatten out into lids. Lay the lid on top of the pies and gently press around the edges to seal. Cut a couple of steam vents in top of each pie.
- Return to the oven for 10-15 minutes until golden brown on top.
- Eat warm, with sugar-free ketchup if you want to feel very Australian. If you can't find sugar-free, you can make your own keto ketchup in just a few minutes!
- Store in the refrigerator for up to 5 days.

Nutrition Info

Net carbs: 2.3g
Protein: 9.9g
Fat: 8.2g
Calories: 123kcal

Healthy scrambled eggs

Scrambled eggs are made extra special by adding smoked salmon. Serve with fresh watercress and grilled vine tomatoes for a more filling breakfast.

Prep time: 30 mins
Cooking time: 10 mins
Serves 2

Ingredients

- 8 midi vine tomatoes, halved
- low-calorie cooking spray
- 3 large free-range eggs
- 35g/1¼oz smoked salmon, roughly chopped
- 1 tbsp chopped chives
- 25g/1oz fresh watercress, to serve
- freshly ground black pepper

Instructions

- Season the tomatoes with pepper. Heat a pan sprayed with cooking oil over a medium heat, add the tomatoes and cook for 2-3 minutes, until softened, stirring from time to time but not breaking up the tomatoes.

- Beat the eggs in a bowl with some pepper. Stir in the salmon and chives and pour into a saucepan.

- Cook very gently for 3-4 minutes, stirring slowly, until the eggs are softly scrambled. Remove from the heat and stir for a few seconds.

- Divide the tomatoes between two plates and serve with the scrambled eggs and watercress.

Nutrition Info

263kcal, 21g protein, 10g carbohydrates (of which 10g sugars), 14g fat (of which 3.5g saturates), 4g fiber and 1g salt.

Moroccan baked eggs

Baked eggs are the perfect dish for a lazy brunch. If you like your eggs spicy, just add a little chilli powder.

Prep time: 30 mins
Cooking time: 10 to 30 mins
Serves 2

Ingredients

- ½ tbsp olive oil
- ½ onion, chopped
- 1 garlic clove, sliced
- ½ tsp ras-el-hanout
- pinch ground cinnamon
- ½ tsp ground coriander
- 400g/14oz cherry tomatoes, chopped
- 2 tbsp chopped coriander
- 2 free-range eggs
- salt and freshly ground black pepper

Instruction

- Preheat the oven to 220C/200C Fan/Gas 7.

- Heat the oil in a frying pan, add the onion and garlic and cook for 6-7 minutes, or until soft. Stir in the spices and cook, stirring, for a further minute.

- Add the tomatoes and season well with salt and pepper, then simmer gently for 8-10 minutes.

- Scatter over 1 tablespoon of the coriander, then divide the tomato mixture between 2 individual ovenproof dishes. Break an egg into each dish.

- Bake for 8-10 minutes until the egg whites are set but the yolks are still slightly runny. Cook for a further 2-3 minutes if you prefer the eggs to be cooked through.

- Scatter over the remaining coriander and serve.

Low-Carb Butter Braised Cabbage with Crispy Ham

Total Time: 2 hours 15 minutes
Serving: 4

Ingredients

- half head white or inexperienced cabbage (600g/1.three lb)
- 2 sticks unsalted butter (225g/8oz)
- sea salt, to style
- black pepper, to style
- 6 slices prosciutto di Parma (90g/ three.2oz)

Instructions

- Slice cabbage and place it in a dutch oven or giant saucepan.

- Chop butter into chunks and sit on prime of cabbage.

- Put lid on pot and prepare dinner on low for about 2 hours, stirring each 15-20 minutes to forestall burning. Don't put water in.

- Warmth oven to 180 °C/ 360 °F (fan assisted). Place prosciutto on a rack over an oven tray and prepare dinner for 10-15 minutes till crispy.

- Cool, then crumble roughly right into a container.

- As soon as cabbage is completed, serve with a wholesome grind of black pepper and crumbled prosciutto on prime.

- Retailer in a container within the fridge for as much as four days.

Vegetables With Red Pepper Rouille

Roasted vegetables do not have to be boring, flavor with saffron and serve with a smoky red pepper rouille to create a tasty vegetarian supper.

Prep time: 30 mins to 1 hour
Cooking time: 30 mins to 1 hour
Serves 6

Ingredients

- 4 tbsp olive oil
- 2-3 garlic cloves, finely chopped
- 3 large pinches of saffron threads
- 3 mixed red and orange peppers, cored, deseeded and each cut into 6 strips
- 3 courgettes, about 100g/3½oz each, chopped into 2.5cm/1in chunks
- 2 onions, cut into wedges
- salt and freshly ground black pepper

For the rouille

- 4 plum tomatoes, about 250g/9oz in total
- 1 red pepper, cored, deseeded and quartered
- 1 garlic clove, finely chopped
- large pinch of ground smoked paprika
- 1 tbsp olive oil

Instruction

- Preheat the oven to 220C/200C Fan/Gas 7.

- Put the oil for the vegetables in a large plastic bag with the garlic, saffron and some salt and pepper. Add the vegetables, grip the top edge of the bag to seal and toss together. Set aside for at least 30 minutes.

- Meanwhile for the rouille, put the tomatoes and pepper in a small roasting tin. Sprinkle with the garlic, smoked paprika some salt and pepper. Then drizzle the oil over and roast for 15 minutes. Allow to cool.

- Peel the skins from the tomatoes and pepper. Purée the flesh in a liquidizer or food processor with any juices from the roasting tin until smooth. Spoon into a serving bowl and set aside, keep warm.

- Tip the saffron vegetables into a large roasting tin and cook in the oven for 15-20 minutes, turning once, until browned.

- Spoon the vegetables on to individual plates and serve with spoonfuls of the rouille.

Nutrition Info

142 kcal per portion.

Garlic Mushroom Frittata

Garlic and mushrooms bring great flavor to this super-low-calorie, easy-to-make frittata. Serve with salad for a simple and delicious lunch.

Prep time: 30 mins
Cooking time: 10 to 30 mins
Serves 2

Ingredients

- low-calorie cooking spray
- 250g/9oz chestnut mushrooms, sliced
- 1 small garlic clove, crushed
- 1 tbsp thinly sliced fresh chives
- 4 large free-range eggs, beaten
- freshly ground black pepper

For the salad

- 1 Little Gem lettuce, leaves separated
- 100g/3½oz cherry tomatoes, halved
- 1/3 cucumber, cut into chunks

Instruction

- Spray a small, flame-proof frying pan with oil and place over a high heat. (The base of the pan shouldn't be wider than about 18cm/7in.) Stir-fry the mushrooms in three batches for 2-3 minutes, or until softened and lightly browned. Tip the cooked mushrooms into a sieve over a bowl to catch any juices – you don't want the mushrooms to become soggy.

- Return all the mushrooms to the pan and stir in the garlic and chives, and a pinch of ground black pepper. Cook for a further minute, then reduce the heat to low.

- Preheat the grill to its hottest setting. Pour the eggs over the mushrooms. Cook for five minutes, or until almost set.

- Place the pan under the grill for 3-4 minutes, or until set.

- Combine the salad ingredients in a bowl.

- Remove from the grill and loosen the sides of the frittata with a round-bladed knife. Turn out onto a board and cut into wedges. Serve hot or cold with the salad.

Nutrition Info

243 kcal, 14g protein, 3.5g carbohydrate (of which 3g sugars), 14g fat (of which 4g saturates), 2.5g fiber and 0.6g salt per portion.

Stir-Fried Pork With Ginger And Soy Sauce

This low-calorie, stir-fried pork is quick and easy while still delivering on flavor, and helping you on your way to getting five a day.

Prep time: 30 mins
Cooking time: 10 to 30 mins
Serves 2

Ingredients

- 250g/9oz pork tenderloin, all visible fat removed, cut into chunks
- 1 tsp cornflour
- 2 tbsp dark soy sauce
- low-calorie cooking spray
- 150g/5½oz button mushrooms, sliced
- 2 red peppers, deseeded and sliced
- 75g/2½oz mangetout, trimmed
- 15g/½oz fresh root ginger, cut into thin matchsticks
- 1 garlic clove, thinly sliced
- 4 spring onions, cut into short lengths
- freshly ground black pepper

Instruction

- Season the pork with pepper. Mix the cornflour with two tablespoons of cold water until smooth, then stir in the soy sauce.

- Spray a large wok, or deep-frying pan, with cooking spray and place over a high heat. Stir-fry the pork for 1-2 minutes, or until lightly browned but not cooked through. Transfer to a plate.

- Return the pan to the heat, reduce the heat a little and spray with more oil. Stir-fry the mushrooms and pepper for 2 minutes. Add the mangetout and cook for a minute. Add the ginger, garlic and spring onions and stir-fry for a few seconds.

- Return the pork to the pan and pour over the soy sauce mixture. Cook for 1-2 minutes, or until the sauce has thickened and the pork is cooked through. Serve immediately.

Salmon BLTs

This delicious high-protein meal comes together in just 20 minutes!

Total Time: 0 hours 20 mins
4 servings

Ingredients

- 8 slices bacon
- ½ c. low-fat Greek yogurt
- ¼ c. dill, chopped
- 1 scallion, finely chopped
- 1 tbsp. oil of choice
- 4 oz. skinless salmon fillet
- 1 tomato, sliced
- romaine lettuce for serving
- toasted bread for serving
- salt and pepper

Instruction

- Working in batches, cook bacon in a large skillet on medium heat until crisp for 5 to 6 minutes; transfer to a paper towel-lined plate.
- Meanwhile, in a bowl, combine low-fat Greek yogurt, chopped dill, finely chopped scallion, and 1/4 tsp each salt and pepper.
- Wipe out the skillet and heat 1 Tbsp oil on medium. Season four 4-oz pieces of skinless salmon fillet with ¼ tsp each salt and pepper and cook until opaque throughout, 1 to 2 minutes per side.

- Spread the yogurt mixture on 4 pieces of bread. Top with romaine lettuce, salmon, 1 sliced tomato, and bacon, then sandwich with another slice of bread.

Nutrition Info

485 calories, 42g protein, 43g carbs, 7g fiber, 10g sugars (6g added sugars), 15g fat (4g sat fat), 72mg cholesterol, 885mg sodium

Italian style meatballs with courgette 'tagliatelle'

This flavourful dish of Italian meatballs has a healthy twist by using courgette ribbons instead of pasta — an easy way to reduce calories.

Prep time: 30 mins
Cooking time: 10 to 30 mins
Serves 2

Ingredients

For the meatballs

- 250g/9oz extra lean beef mince (5% fat or less)
- 1 small onion, very finely chopped
- 1 tsp dried mixed herbs
- calorie controlled cooking oil spray
- 1 garlic clove, crushed
- 227g/8oz can chopped tomatoes
- 2 heaped tbsp finely shredded fresh basil leaves, plus extra to garnish

For the courgette 'tagliatelle'

- 2 medium courgettes, trimmed and deseeded
- sea salt and freshly ground black pepper

Instructions

- Place the beef, half the onion, half the mixed herbs and a pinch of salt and pepper in a bowl and mix well. Form into 10 small balls.

- Spray a medium non-stick frying pan with a little oil and cook the meatballs for 5-7 minutes, turning occasionally until browned on all sides. Transfer to a plate.

- For the sauce, put the remaining onion in the same pan and cook over a low heat for three minutes, stirring. Add the garlic and cook for a few seconds.

- Stir in the tomatoes, 300ml/10fl oz water, the remaining mixed herbs and shredded basil. Bring to the boil, stirring. Return the meatballs to the pan, reduce the heat to a simmer and cook for 20 minutes, stirring occasionally until the sauce is thick and the meatballs are cooked throughout.

- Meanwhile, half-fill a medium pan with water and bring to the boil. Use a vegetable peeler to peel the courgettes into ribbons. Cook the courgette in the boiling water for one minute then drain.

- Divide the courgette ribbons between two plates and top with the meatballs and sauce. Garnish with basil leaves.

Nutrition Info

219 kcal per portion.

Chilli And Coriander Fish Parcel

Baking fish is a great way to reduce calories. Give the fish extra oomph with chilli and coriander.

Prep time: 1-2 hours
Cooking time: 10 to 30 mins
Serves 1

Ingredients

- 125g/4½oz cod, coley or haddock fillet
- 2 tsp lemon juice
- 1 tbsp fresh coriander leaves
- 1 garlic clove, roughly chopped
- 1 green chilli, deseeded and chopped
- ¼ tsp sugar
- 2 tsp natural yogurt
- 80g/3oz mangetout, steamed, to serve

Instruction

- Preheat the oven to 200C/180C Fan/Gas 6.

- Place the fish in a non-metallic dish and sprinkle with the lemon juice. Cover and leave in the fridge to marinate for 15-20 minutes.

- Put the coriander, garlic and chilli in a food processor or blender and process until the mixture forms a paste. Add the sugar and yoghurt and briefly process to blend.

- Lay the fish on a sheet of foil. Coat the fish on both sides with the paste. Gather up the foil loosely and turn over at the top to seal. Return to the fridge for at least 1 hour.

- Place the parcel on a baking tray and bake for about 15 minutes, or until the fish is just cooked. Serve with the mangetout.

Extra-Lean Burger And Salad

Prep time: 30 mins
Cooking time: 10 to 30 mins
Serves 2

Ingredients

- low-calorie cooking spray
- ½ small onion, finely chopped
- 100g/3½oz Portobello mushrooms, finely chopped
- 250g/9oz extra-lean beef mince (under 5% fat)
- 2 tsp finely chopped fresh thyme (or ½ tsp dried thyme)
- freshly ground black pepper

For the salad

- 1 Little Gem lettuce, leaves separated
- 120g/4½oz cherry tomatoes, sliced
- 1/3 cucumber, sliced

Instruction

- Spray a small frying pan with oil and cook the onion and mushrooms over a medium heat for five minutes, or until well softened, stirring regularly. Tip into a heatproof bowl and leave to cool for five minutes.

- Add the beef, thyme and lots of ground black pepper. Mix well and form into two balls. Flatten into burger shapes, each around 2cm/¾in thick.

- Clean the pan and return to the hob. Spray with a little more oil and cook the burgers over a medium-low heat for 10 minutes, turning occasionally, until browned on the outside and cooked through inside.

- Serve the burgers with lettuce, tomatoes and cucumber.

Nutrition Info

255 kcal, 36g protein, 6g carbohydrate (of which 5.5g sugars), 7g fat (of which 2.5g saturates), 3g fiber and 0.4g salt per portion.

Red mullet with baked tomatoes

Prep time: 30 mins
Cooking time: 10 to 30 mins
Serves 4

Ingredients

For the tomatoes

- 375g/13oz mixed red and yellow cherry tomatoes
- 320g/11½oz fine green beans, trimmed
- 2 garlic cloves, finely chopped
- 2 tbsp lemon juice
- low-calorie cooking spray
- salt and freshly ground black pepper

For the red mullet

- 8 red mullet fillets, approximately 100g/3½oz each
- 1 lemon, finely grated rind only
- 2 tsp baby capers, drained
- 2 spring onions, finely sliced

To garnish

- 2 tbsp chopped parsley
- 8 caperberries

Instruction

- Preheat the oven to 200C/180C Fan/Gas 6.

- Put the tomatoes in an ovenproof dish with the beans, garlic, lemon juice and spray with the oil. Season with salt and freshly ground black pepper and mix well. Bake for 10 minutes, or until the tomatoes and beans are tender.

- Meanwhile, tear off 4 large sheets of foil and line with non-stick baking paper. Place 2 fish fillets on each piece of baking paper, then scatter over the lemon rind, capers and spring onions, season with salt and freshly ground black pepper. Fold over the paper-lined foil and scrunch the edges together to seal. Place the parcels on a large baking tray.

- Place the fish parcels next to the vegetables in the oven and bake for a further 8-10 minutes, or until the flesh flakes easily when pressed in the centre with a knife.

- Spoon the vegetables on to four serving plates and top each with two fish fillets. Garnish with the parsley and caperberries and serve.

Nutrition Info

248 kcal.

Chicken And Vegetable Balti

Try this chicken and vegetable balti for a healthy curry that is quick and easy to prepare.

Prep time: 30 mins
Cooking time: 30 mins to 1 hour
Serves 2

Ingredients

- calorie controlled cooking oil spray
- 1 medium onion, thinly sliced
- 4 chicken thighs, boned and skinned
- 1 red pepper, deseeded and cut into 3cm/1in chunks
- 1 yellow pepper, deseeded and cut into 3cm/1in chunks
- 1 tbsp cornflour
- 150g/5½oz fat-free natural yogurt
- 1 tbsp medium or mild curry powder
- 2 garlic cloves, thinly sliced
- 227g/8oz tin chopped tomatoes
- 3 heaped tbsp finely chopped fresh coriander, plus extra to garnish
- freshly ground black pepper

Instructions

- Spray a large, deep, non-stick frying pan or wok with oil and place over a medium heat. Add the onion and cook for five minutes, stirring regularly until well softened and lightly browned.

- Meanwhile, trim all the visible fat off the chicken thighs, cut each one into four pieces and season with black pepper.

- Add the chicken and peppers into the pan with the onion and cook for three minutes, turning occasionally.

- Meanwhile, in a small bowl, mix the cornflour with 2 tablespoons cold water and stir in the yoghurt until thoroughly mixed.

- Sprinkle the curry powder over the chicken and vegetables, add the garlic and cook for 30 seconds.

- Tip the tomatoes into the pan, add the yogurt mixture, 150ml/3½fl oz of water and coriander.

- Bring to a gentle simmer and cook for 20-25 minutes, stirring occasionally until the chicken is tender and the sauce is thick. Season with freshly ground black pepper to taste and garnish with coriander.

Nutrition Info

341 kcal, 40g protein, 30.5g carbohydrate (of which 20.5g sugars), 6g fat (of which 1.5g saturates), 9g fiber and 0.6g salt per portion.

Poached Eggs With Bacon And Tomatoes

A great alternative to the traditional fry-up that's low in calories but high in flavour. Poached eggs are a great way to make breakfast a little lighter and surprisingly easy to cook.

Prep time: 30 mins
Cooking time: less than 10 mins
Serves 2

Ingredients

2 large ripe tomatoes, halved
4 rashers smoked back bacon, all visible fat removed
2 medium free-range eggs
ground black pepper

Instruction

- Preheat the grill to its hottest setting. Put the tomatoes on a rack over a grill pan lined with foil. Season with pepper.

- Grill for 3 minutes, then add the bacon and grill for a further 4 minutes, turning the bacon after 2 minutes so that it is lightly browned on both sides.

- Meanwhile, half-fill a medium pan with water and bring it to the boil. Crack the eggs into two small bowls. Turn the heat down so that the water is bubbling very gently. Slowly add the eggs to the water and cook for 3 minutes or until the white is set but the yolk remains runny.

- Using a slotted spoon, scoop the eggs out of the water and divide between two plates. Add the cooked bacon and tomatoes. Season with a little salt and pepper and serve.

Peppered Beef With Salad Leaves

This is a speedy supper, perfect for a busy evening. Horseradish sauce adds a kick to the salad dressing.

Prep time: 30 mins
Cooking time: less than 10 mins
Serves 2

Ingredients

- 2 thick-cut sirloin steaks, about 175g/6oz in total, fat trimmed
- 1 tsp coloured peppercorns, coarsely crushed
- coarse salt flakes
- 60g/2¼oz natural yogurt
- ½ tsp horseradish sauce (to taste)
- ½ garlic clove, crushed
- 50g/2oz mixed green salad leaves
- 30g/1¼oz button mushrooms, sliced
- ½ red onion, thinly sliced
- 1 tsp olive oil
- salt and freshly ground black pepper

Instructions

- Rub the steaks with the crushed peppercorns and salt flakes.

- Mix the yogurt, horseradish sauce and garlic and season to taste with salt and freshly ground black pepper. Add the salad leaves, mushrooms and most of the red onion and toss gently.

- Heat the oil in a frying pan, add the steaks and cook over a high heat for 2 minutes, or until browned. Turn over and cook for a further 2 minutes for medium rare, 3-4 minutes for medium or 5 minutes for well done. Place the steak on a warm plate and allow to rest for a few minutes.

- Spoon the salad leaves into the center of 2 serving plates. Thinly slice the steaks and arrange the pieces on top. Garnish with the remaining red onion.

Nutrition Info

148 kcal

Lamb And Flageolet Bean Stew

This is a warming stew perfect for filling you up on a cold evening. Don't be put off by the long cooking time, this is an easy one-pot supper that will reward you for your patience.

Prep time: 30 mins
Cooking time: 1 to 2 hours
Serves 4

Ingredients

- 1 tsp olive oil
- 350g/12oz lean lamb, cubed
- 16 pickling onions
- 1 garlic clove, crushed
- 600ml/20fl oz lamb stock (made with concentrated liquid stock)
- 200g can of chopped tomatoes
- 1 bouquet garni
- 2 x 400g cans flageolet beans, drained and rinsed
- 320g/11oz green beans
- 250g/9oz cherry tomatoes
- freshly ground black pepper

Instruction

- Heat the oil in a flameproof casserole or saucepan, add the lamb and fry for 3-4 minutes until browned all over. Remove the lamb from the casserole and set aside.

- Add the onions and garlic to the pan and fry for 4-5 minutes, or until the onions are beginning to brown.

- Return the lamb and any juices to the pan. Add the stock, tomatoes, bouquet garni and beans. Bring to the boil, stirring, then cover and simmer for 1 hour, or until the lamb is just tender.

- Meanwhile, bring a pan of water to the boil and blanch the green beans. Place in a bowl of ice-cold water.

- Add the cherry tomatoes to the stew and season well with freshly ground black pepper. Continue to simmer for 10 minutes.

- Divide the stew between four plates, place the green beans alongside and serve.

Nutrition Info

288 kcal per portion.

Chermoula Tofu And Roasted Vegetables

Tofu wonderfully absorbs the flavours of chermoula in this dish. Serve with roasted vegetables for a hearty vegetarian meal.

As part of an Intermittent diet plan, 1 serving provides 2 of your 6 daily vegetable portions. This meal provides 182 kcal per portion.

Prep time: 30 mins
Cooking time: 30 mins to 1 hour
Serves 4

Ingredients

For the chermoula tofu

- 25g/1oz coriander, finely chopped
- 3 garlic cloves, chopped
- 1 tsp cumin seeds, lightly crushed
- 1 lemon, finely grated rind
- ½ tsp dried crushed chillies
- 1 tbsp olive oil
- 250g/9oz tofu

For the roasted vegetables

- 2 red onions, quartered
- 2 courgettes, thickly sliced
- 2 red peppers, deseeded and sliced
- 2 yellow peppers, deseeded and sliced
- 1 small aubergine, thickly sliced
- low-calorie cooking spray
- pinch salt

Instruction

- Preheat the oven to 200C/180C Fan/Gas 6.

- For the chermoula, mix the coriander, garlic, cumin, lemon rind and chilies together with the oil and a little salt in a small bowl.

- Pat the tofu dry on kitchen paper and cut it in half. Cut each half horizontally into thin slices. Spread the chermoula generously over the slices.

- Scatter the vegetables in a roasting tin and spray with oil. Bake for about 45 minutes, until lightly browned, turning the ingredients once or twice during cooking.

- Arrange the tofu slices over the vegetables, with the side spread with the chermoula uppermost, and bake for a further 10-15 minutes, or until the tofu is lightly coloured.

- Divide the tofu and vegetables between four plates and serve.

Hearty Vegetable Soup

This hearty vegetable soup is packed full of flavor and goodness, perfect to warm you up on a cold night.

Prep time: 30 mins
Cooking time: 30 mins to 1 hour
Serves 2

Ingredients

- calorie controlled cooking oil spray
- 1 medium onion, sliced
- 2 garlic cloves, thinly sliced
- 2 celery sticks, trimmed and thinly sliced
- 2 medium carrots or 2 yellow peppers, cut into 2cm/1in chunks
- 400g/14oz tin chopped tomatoes
- 1 vegetable stock cube
- 1 tsp dried mixed herbs
- 400g/14oz tin butter beans, drained and rinsed
- 1 head young spring greens (approximately 125g/4½oz), trimmed and sliced
- sea salt and freshly ground black pepper

Instructions

- Spray a large non-stick saucepan with oil and cook the onion, garlic, celery and carrots or peppers gently for 10 minutes, stirring regularly until softened.

- Add 750ml/26fl oz water and the chopped tomatoes. Crumble over the stock cube and stir in the dried herbs. Bring to the boil, then reduce the heat to a simmer and cook for 20 minutes.

- Season the soup with salt and pepper and add the spring greens and butterbeans. Return to a gentle simmer and cook for a further 3-4 minutes or until the greens are softened. Season to taste and serve in deep bowls.

Nutrition Info

219 kcal per portion.

Caponata Ratatouille

Ratatouille is a wonderfully warming vegetable stew originating from Provence. Perfect for pleasing vegetarians and meat-eaters alike.

Prep time: 30 mins
Cooking time: 30 mins to 1 hour
Serves 6

Ingredients

- 1 tbsp olive oil
- 750g/1lb 10oz aubergines, cut into 1cm/1½in chunks
- 1 large onion, cut into 1cm/1½in chunks
- 3 celery sticks, roughly chopped
- 2 large beef tomatoes, skinned and deseeded
- 1 tsp chopped thyme
- ¼-½ tsp cayenne pepper
- 2 tbsp capers, drained
- small handful pitted green olives
- 4 tbsp white wine vinegar
- 1 tbsp sugar
- 1-2 tbsp cocoa powder (optional)
- freshly ground black pepper
- To garnish
- chopped almonds, toasted
- chopped parsley

Instructions

- Heat the oil in a non-stick frying pan until very hot, add the aubergine and fry for about 15 minutes, or until very soft. Add a little boiling water to prevent sticking if necessary.

- Meanwhile, place the onion and celery in a large saucepan with a little water. Cook for 5 minutes, or until tender but still firm.

- Add the tomatoes, thyme, cayenne pepper and aubergine to the saucepan. Cook for 15 minutes, stirring occasionally. Add the capers, olives, vinegar, sugar and cocoa powder and cook for 2-3 minutes.

- Season with freshly ground black pepper. Divide between 6 bowls, garnish with the toasted almonds and parsley and serve.

Italian Omelet

This omelet is simply delicious with fresh tomato, basil, and Land O Lakes® Eggs!

10 min Prep Time
20 min Total Time
2 servings

Ingredients

Topping

- 1 medium (½ cup) tomato, seeded, chopped
- 2 tablespoons sliced green onion
- 1 tablespoon chopped fresh basil leaves

Eggs

- 1 tablespoon Land O Lakes® Butter
- 1 teaspoon finely chopped fresh garlic
- 4 large Land O Lakes® Eggs
- 1 tablespoon water or milk
- ¼ teaspoon salt
- 1/8 teaspoon pepper
- ½ cup shredded mozzarella cheese
- 2 tablespoons shredded Parmesan cheese

Instruction

- Combine all topping ingredients in bowl; set aside.
- Melt butter in 10-inch nonstick skillet over medium heat until sizzling. Add garlic; cook 1 minute.
- Beat eggs, water, salt and pepper in bowl at low speed until light in color and well mixed. Pour eggs into hot skillet.

Cook 2 minutes; lift edge of eggs with heat proof spatula to allow uncooked portion to flow underneath 3-4 minutes or until mixture is almost set.

- Sprinkle mozzarella cheese over half of omelet. Cover; let stand 1-2 minutes or until cheese is melted. Gently fold other half of omelet over cheese.

- Place omelet onto plate; top with Parmesan cheese and tomato mixture. Cut in half.

Nutrition Info

310 Calories
23 Fat (g)
455 Cholesterol (mg)
720 Sodium (mg)
4 Carbohydrates (g)
1 Dietary Fiber
21 Protein (g)

Keto Crispy Ginger Mackerel Lunch Bowl

This recipe takes mackerel and turns it into a flavor-packed meal. We marinate the fish in ginger, lemon, and coconut aminos before roasting it in the oven. The base of the bowl is broccoli, sun-dried tomatoes, and peppers. Then everything is finished off with roasted almonds and guac.

Servings: 2

Ingredients

Marinade:

- 1 tablespoon grated ginger
- 1 tablespoon lemon juice
- 3 tablespoons olive oil
- 1 tablespoon coconut aminos
- Salt and pepper, to taste

Lunch bowl:

- 2 (8-ounce) boneless mackerel fillets
- 1-ounce almonds
- 1 ½ cups broccoli
- 1 tablespoon butter
- ½ small yellow onion
- 1/3 cup diced red bell pepper
- 2 small sun-dried tomatoes, chopped
- 4 tablespoons mashed avocado

Instruction

- Preheat the oven to 400 °F. Line a baking tray with parchment paper or foil. Mix together the grated ginger, lemon juice, olive oil, coconut aminos, and some salt and pepper. Rub half of the marinade on the mackerel fillets.

- Lay the fillets onto the baking tray with the skin side facing up. Roast for 12-15 minutes or until the skin is crispy.

- Spread the almonds out on a separate baking sheet. Roast for 5-6 minutes or until they brown. Take out of the oven and cool before chopping.

- Lightly steam the broccoli until it's started to soften but isn't mushy. Roughly chop it up.

- Preheat a pan over medium heat, then add the butter and allow it to melt. Fry the onions and peppers until they are soft.

- Add the broccoli and sun-dried tomatoes, then continue cooking until warmed through.

- Turn off the heat then mix in the rest of the dressing and roasted almonds. Serve with the avocado.

Nutrition Info

649.55 Calories, 53.4g Fats, 9.2g Net Carbs, and 28.05g Protein.

Smoked Salmon, Avocado & Egg Lunch Bowl

A delicious smoked salmon and avocado recipe optimised for a healthy ketogenic diet. Topped with a perfect soft poached egg and my favorite 2 minute avocado smash. It's the perfect dish for those who practice intermittent fasting and only eat two nutritious meals a day. It's high in healthy omega 3 fats, it's a fantastic source of protein, and one serving will cover more than half of your daily magnesium and potassium.

Servings: 1

Ingredients

Salad:

- 2 tbsp pumpkin seeds (16g/0.6oz)
- 1 tsp sesame seeds
- ½ large avocado (100g/3.5oz)
- 1 tsp lime or lemon juice
- 1 tsp extra virgin olive oil
- 1/8 tsp chile flakes
- pinch of salt and pepper
- 1 small head crispy lettuce such as baby gem (100g/3.5oz)
- 1 large egg
- 150g smoked salmon (5.3oz)

To Serve:

- 2 tbsp extra virgin olive oil (30ml)
- 1 tbsp lemon juice (15ml)
- pinch of salt and pepper
- 1 tbsp butter, ghee or bacon grease (14g/0.5oz)
- 1 tsp paprika

- 2 tbsp full-fat Greek yogurt or paleo mayonnaise (30g/1.1oz)

Instructions

- Preheat the oven to 180 °C/ 355 °F (fan assisted) 200 °C/ 400 °F (conventional). Place the seeds on a baking tray and roast for 8 minutes until golden. Remove from the oven and allow to cool. Alternatively, roast on a hot dry pan for a few minutes until the pumpkin seeds puff up.
- Place the peeled and pitted avocado into a bowl and smash using a fork. Mix all the smashed avocado ingredients together in a small bowl. Add lime juice, olive oil, chile flakes, salt and pepper and mix well.
- In a separate bowl, mix the dressing ingredients together.
- Poach the eggs by filling a saucepan full of boiling water from the kettle. Bring to a light simmer over a medium heat and season with salt.
- Crack each egg into a cup one at a time. Swirl the water gently with a spoon in a circular direction and carefully pour the egg into the water. Cook for about 3 (soft) - 5 minutes (hard). Remove with a slotted spoon and place on kitchen paper to drain. Smoked Salmon, Avocado & Egg Lunch Bowl.
- Melt the butter in a pan on a low heat. Once melted, add the paprika and immediately turn off the heat. Do not let the butter burn or it will discolor it. Allow to cool slightly. Place yogurt in a bowl and swirl through paprika butter.
- Place the baby gem lettuce leaves in your serving bowl.
- Top with smoked salmon, dressing, toasted seeds, smashed avocado, chilli flakes and paprika butter yogurt.
- Top with the poached egg. Tastes best when served fresh but can be stored in the fridge for up to a day.

Nutrition Info

Net carbs: 7.7 grams
Protein: 45 grams
Fat: 80.7 grams
Calories: 949 kcal

Speedy Low-Carb Tuna Lunch Bowl

This speedy, low-carb lunch bowl is the perfect balance of protein, healthy fats and is low in net carbs. Ready in just 15 minutes, it's one of my favourite go to healthy gluten-free and keto-friendly meals. It's the ideal dish for those who practice intermittent fasting and only eat two nutritious meals a day.

Prep/Cook Time: 15 minutes
Servings: 3

Ingredients

- 1 tuna steak (120g/4.2oz) - or use tinned, drained tuna
- 1 tsp sesame seeds
- pinch of sea salt
- 1 tsp ghee, butter or virgin coconut oil
- ½ avocado, sliced (100g/3.5oz)
- 10 pitted black olives (30g/1.1oz)
- 1 tbsp mayonnaise (15g/0.5oz) - you can make your own mayo
- ½ medium cucumber, sliced (70g/2.5oz)
- 6 ⍰uails eggs or 1 large egg
- ¼ small red onion, finely sliced (15g/0.5oz)
- 10 walnut halves (20g/0.7oz)
- 1 tbsp extra virgin olive oil (15ml)
- large handful of watercress (50g/1.8oz)

Instructions

- Preheat the oven to 180 °C/ 355 °F (fan assisted) 200 °C/ 400 °F (conventional). Wash and dry the watercress.

- Place the walnuts on a baking tray and roast in the oven for 6-8 minutes until golden. Remove from the oven and allow to cool.
- Coat the tuna with sesame seeds, ghee and a pinch of salt. If using tinned tuna, simply sprinkle the sesame seeds over the salad in the end.
- Heat a griddle pan and fry the tuna to your liking - 1 ½ minutes per side for pink, up to 3 minutes per side for well done. Remove from the heat and allow to cool slightly before slicing.
- Boil the quail eggs for 2-3 minutes (or about 10 minutes for large eggs). Plunge into cold water before peeling.
- Slice the rest of ingredients.
- Place the watercress in bowl and add olives, halved quail eggs, avocado, walnuts and drizzle with 1 tbsp of olive oil and top with 1 tbsp of mayonnaise. Optionally, garnish with ground black pepper.
- Tastes the best when served fresh, but can be stored in the fridge for 1 day.

Nutrition Info

Net carbs: 6.4g
Protein: 44.2g
Fat: 71.3g
Calories: 866 kcal

Low-Carb Veggie Full English Breakfast Bowl

Prep/Cook Time: 35 minutes
Servings: 1

Ingredients

- 3 red, yellow or orange baby peppers or 1 small bell pepper (60g/2.1oz)
- 1 tsp ghee or extra virgin olive oil
- pinch of sea salt, to taste
- 1 tsp pumpkin seeds
- 1 tsp sunflower seeds
- 1 tsp flax seeds
- 1 tbsp butter, ghee or extra virgin olive oil (15ml)
- ¾ cup shredded kale or spinach (38g/1.3oz)
- 1/3 cup sliced shiitake or white mushrooms (25g/0.9oz)
- 3 slices halloumi cheese (50g/1.8oz)
- 1 tsp ghee or extra virgin olive oil
- 1 tbsp homemade Low-Carb Marinara Sauce (15ml)
- few basil leaves

Smashed avocado:

- ½ small avocado (75g/2.7oz)
- 1 tsp fresh lime juice
- 1 tsp extra virgin olive oil
- pinch of sea salt and black pepper, to taste
- 1/8 tsp chile flakes

Instructions

- Preheat the oven to 180 °C/ 355 °F (fan assisted) or 200 °C/ 400 °F (conventional). Place the peppers on a baking tray

- and drizzle with olive oil and a pinch of salt. Roast in the oven for 25 minutes until soft.
- Place the seeds on another baking tray and roast in the oven for 4 minutes until golden. Remove from the oven and allow to cool.
- Note: You can make a large batch of the roasted seeds and keep at room temperature for up to 2 weeks, ready to be used for topping or snacking.
- Heat the butter on a medium heat in a non-stick pan, add the mushrooms and cook for 2 minutes. Add the kale and cook for a further 2 minutes. Season with a pinch of salt to taste.
- Fry the halloumi in 1 tsp of ghee or olive oil over a medium-low heat for about 2 minutes per side, or until golden.
- Once the peppers are cooked, allow to cool slightly. Remove the stalks and scoop out the seeds.
- Smash the avocado with a fork and mix with the olive oil, salt, pepper, lime and chile flakes.
- Place the kale and mushrooms in your bowl, along with the seeds, peppers, halloumi and top with smashed avocado, marinara sauce and fresh basil.
- 8 Best served fresh. The cooked vegetables can be stored in a sealed jar in the fridge for up to 3 days and served warm or cold. Halloumi should always be reheated before serving.

Nutrition Info

Net carbs: 9.7 grams
Protein: 15.9 grams
Fat: 60.7 grams
Calories: 662 kcal

Low-Carb Chocolate Coconut Smoothie

Low-carb smoothies like this chocolate coconut smoothie is a healthy breakfast option for busy mornings. Thanks to healthy fats from avocado and coconut cream, this keto smoothie will keep you full until lunch. Avocado and cacao are high in electrolytes, especially magnesium and potassium, and will keep keto flu at bay. You can optionally add collagen, whipped cream and cocoa nibs. Enjoy!

Prep/Cook Time: 5 minutes
Servings: 2

Ingredients

Smoothie:

- ½ large avocado (100g/3.5oz)
- 1 ¼ cup almond milk (300ml/10fl oz)
- ¼ cup coconut cream or heavy whipping cream (60ml/2fl oz)
- 1 tbsp flax meal or chia seeds (7g/0.3oz)
- 1 ½ tbsp cacao powder (8g/0.3oz)
- 1 tsp virgin coconut oil or MCT oil
- 1 heaped tbsp almond butter, or other nut or seed butter) (32g/1.1oz)
- Optional: water if too thick

Optional extras:

- 1-2 tbsp collagen for extra protein boost
- healthy low-carb sweetener, to taste

- 1-2 tbsp whipped cream for topping
- 1 tsp cacao nibs or chopped dark chocolate for topping

Instructions

- Place all the ingredients in a high speed blender and blitz until smooth.
- Pour the fat burning keto smoothie into a glass and serve. If using whipped cream for topping: Whip the coconut or heavy whipping cream using a hand blender until thick. Optionally, add cocoa nibs or chopped dark chocolate.
- Best served fresh but can be stored in the fridge for 1 day. Low-Carb Chocolate Coconut Smoothie

Nutrition Info

Net carbs: 6.8 grams
Protein: 12.4 grams
Fat: 42.8 grams
Calories: 510 kcal

Healthy Salmon & Tabbouleh Low-Carb Bowl

If you prefer to have two large meals a day rather than three regular ones, or you've been exercising, this keto-friendly Salmon Bowl with Tabbouleh is the perfect dish for you. It's also one of my favorite meals to break a fast with if you've been practicing intermittent fasting. I much prefer to eat this way than little and often. Carb up keto meals really work for me.

Prep/Cook Time: 30 minutes
Servings: 2

Ingredients

Salmon & tabbouleh bowl:

- 2 medium salmon fillet (300g/10.6oz)
- sea salt and black pepper, to taste
- 1 tbsp extra olive oil or ghee (15ml)
- ½ small cauliflower (240g/ 8.5oz) - will make 2 cups of cauliflower rice
- ½ cup shredded red cabbage (35g/1.2oz)
- ¼ cup chopped sugar snap peas (25g/0.9oz)
- 1/3 cup chopped red pepper (50g/ 1.8oz)
- ¼ small red onion, finely sliced (15g/0.5oz)
- Optional: 1 tbsp pomegranate seeds (5g/0.2oz)
- ¼ cup chopped fresh parsley (15g/0.5oz)
- 2 tbsp chopped fresh mint
- ½ cup crumbled feta (75g/2.7oz)
- 3 tbsp olive oil (45ml)
- 2 tsp fresh lemon juice

Basil yogurt dressing

- 1 heaped tbsp full-fat 5% Greek yogurt (30g/ 1.1oz)

- 1 tbsp chopped fresh basil
- 1 tsp fresh lemon juice
- sea salt and black pepper, to taste

Instructions

- Preheat the oven to 180 °C/ 350 °F (fan assisted) or 200 °C/ 400 °F (conventional). Line a baking tray with greaseproof paper. Season the salmon with salt, pepper and 1 tsp of olive oil. Place on the tray (skin side up) and roast in the oven for 25 minutes until cooked through and the skin is crisp. Option to pan fry if you prefer.
- Blitz the cauliflower florets using the S blade or a grating blade of your food processor until it resembles a rice size consistency.
- Place in a bowl and microwave on high for 4 minutes. Remove from the microwave and allow to cool. (Option to transfer to a muslin cloth and squeeze out the excess water.) This makes it fluffier. Fluff with a fork.
- Mix the olive oil, lemon, salt and pepper together in a small bowl.
- Healthy Salmon & Tabbouleh Low-Carb Bowl
- Add the chopped red cabbage, sugar snap peas, red onion, red pepper, fresh herbs (plus optionally add pomegranate seeds). Add the olive oil dressing and half of the feta to the cooled cauliflower rice. Toss to combine.
- Mix the basil yogurt dressing ingredients together in a small bowl. Place the tabbouleh in your serving bowl.
- Top with roast salmon, the remaining feta and basil yogurt dressing.
- Best fresh but can be stored in the fridge for 3 days.
- Healthy Salmon & Tabbouleh Low-Carb Bowl

Nutrition Info

Net carbs: 9.6 grams

Protein: 42.8 grams
Fat: 45.2 grams
Calories: 629 kcal

Bacon, Egg & Asparagus Keto Bowl

This simple, fresh keto salad takes the American's favorite combination of bacon and eggs to a whole new level. Just one serving is nutritious enough to be part of any keto meal plan that includes intermittent fasting (if you're eating just twice a day).

Prep/Cook Time: 20-25 minutes
Servings: 2

Ingredients

- 4 slices raw bacon (120g/4.2oz) - or 64g/2.2oz crisped up
- 10-14 asparagus spears, woody ends removed (100g/3.5oz)
- 1 tbsp butter or ghee (14g/0.5oz)
- 2 large eggs
- 1 small head lettuce such as little gem (100g/3.5oz)
- ½ large avocado, sliced (100g/3.5oz)
- 1/3 cup crumpled feta cheese (50g/1.8oz)
- 1/3 cup cherry tomatoes, halved (50g/1.8oz)
- 2 tsp chopped chives or spring onion
- ¼ cup flaked almonds, preferably toasted (23g/0.8oz)

DRESSING

- 3 tbsp extra virgin olive oil (45ml/1.5fl oz)
- 1 tsp Dijon mustard
- 2 tsp red wine vinegar
- sea salt and black pepper, to taste

Instructions

- Crisp up the bacon in the oven or in a skillet. Oven is better for large batches. If you're only cooking 4 slices it's faster to cook in a lightly greased skillet.
- Skillet: In a frying pan, fry the bacon rashers for 2 minutes per side until crisp. I dry fried them but you can add a touch of olive oil or ghee if you prefer to prevent sticking. All depends on your pan. Drain on a sheet of kitchen paper.
- Oven: Preheat the oven to 190 °C/ 375 °F. Line a baking tray with baking paper. Lay the bacon strips out flat on the baking paper, leaving space so they don't overlap. Place the tray in the oven and cook for about 10-15 minutes until golden brown. The time depends on the thickness of the bacon slices. When done, remove from the oven and set aside to cool down. Store any leftover bacon in the fridge for up to 4 days.
- Slice the tomatoes and avocado. Chop the lettuce. Bacon, Egg & Asparagus Keto Bowl
- Prepare the dressing my mixing the olive oil, mustard, vinegar, salt and pepper together in a small bowl.
- Place water in the bottom of a steamer pan. Steam the asparagus for 5 – 8 minutes depending on the thickness of the asparagus until el dente. Remove from the pan, coat in 1 tablespoon of butter and chop into chunks.
- While the asparagus is cooking, boil the eggs to your liking. 3 minutes for soft boiled up to 10 minutes for hard boiled. Run under cold water before peeling off the shell.
- Toss the lettuce through the tomatoes, crispy bacon and dressing. Top with boiled egg, feta, avocado, asparagus, chives, and almonds.
- Best eaten fresh but can be stored in the fridge for a day.

Nutrition Info

Net carbs: 5.3 grams
Protein: 25 grams
Fat: 53.4 grams
Calories: 609 kcal

Easy Pork Chops With Asparagus and Hollandaise

Prep/Cook Time: 20-25 minutes
Servings: 3

Ingredients

- ½ cup butter, ghee or extra virgin olive oil (120ml/4fl oz)
- 3 large egg yolks
- 1 tbsp lemon juice (15ml)
- 3 pork loin chops, bone in (200g/7.1oz each), or use 3 boneless pork chops (150g/5.3oz each)
- 2 tbsp ghee or lard (30g/1.1oz)
- 300 g asparagus spears (10.6oz)
- salt and pepper, to taste

Instructions

- Prepare the one-minute Hollandaise. Place ½ cup butter or ghee into a wide mouthed jar, with enough room for a handheld blender to fit into. Melt the butter in the microwave.
- Add the egg yolks and the lemon juice. Place the hand blender in the bottom of the jar and blitz until well combined, lifting it slowly as you blend. Taste and season, if re?uired.
- Heat a frying pan over med-high heat and melt the remaining ghee. Cook the pork chops for 6 minutes on each side and then rest for 5 minutes.
- Meanwhile, bring a pot of water to the boil and then blanch the asparagus for 5 minutes. Remove from the water and drain well.
- Serve pork chops with asparagus spears placed over them, and then drizzle the hollandaise over the top.

- Store the pork and asparagus in the refrigerator, wrapped for 2 days.
- Store the hollandaise in its jar, with the lid on, in the refrigerator for 4 days, warming it before use.

Note:

If a recipe calls for raw eggs and you are concerned about the potential risk of Salmonella, you can make it safe by using pasteurized eggs. To pasteurize eggs at home, simply pour enough water in a saucepan to cover the eggs. Heat to about 60 °C/140 °F. Using a spoon, slowly place the eggs into the saucepan. Keep the eggs in the water for about 3 minutes. This should be enough to pasteurize the eggs and kill any potential bacteria. Let the eggs cool down and store in the fridge for 6-8 weeks.

Nutrition Info

Net carbs: 2.8 grams
Protein: 36 grams
Fat: 58.8 grams
Calories: 690 kcal

Low-Carb All Day Mexican Bowl

This healthy Mexican nourish bowl is super easy to make and packed full of flavor. Low in carbs and high in healthy fats to keep you fuller for longer and your insulin levels stable.

Prep/Cook Time: 20-25 minutes
Servings: 2

Ingredients

- 2 Mexican chorizo sausages (160g/5.6oz)
- 2 gluten-free Italian style sausages (160g/5.6oz)
- ½ jalapeno pepper (7g/0.3oz)
- 1 tbsp fresh oregano or 1 tsp dried oregano
- 1 small yellow onion, diced (45g/1.6oz)
- ½ cup halved cherry tomatoes (75g/2.6oz)
- ½ red bell pepper, chopped (60g/2.1oz)
- 1 medium spring onion, sliced (15g/0.5oz)
- 1 tbsp extra virgin olive oil (15ml)
- ¼ tsp coconut aminos
- 1 tsp fresh lime juice
- 1 tbsp chopped fresh coriander
- 2 large eggs
- ½ large avocado, sliced (100g/3.5oz)
- ¼ tsp paprika
- salt and pepper, to taste

Optional extras:

- few tortilla chips made from Keto Tortillas
- dollop of sour cream

- 1-2 tsp Sriracha sauce (you can make your own fermented sriracha)

Instructions

- Remove the casing from the Italian sausage and chorizo. Fry the meat in a dry, non-stick pan, for 5 minutes breaking it up as you fry so it resembles a mince consistency, until browned.
- Add the onion, paprika and jalapeño and fry on a medium / low heat for 6 – 8 minutes until the onion is soft and translucent. Set aside.
- In a bowl, mix the olive oil, lime, coconut aminos and a pinch of salt and pepper in a bowl. Toss with the tomatoes, oregano, red pepper and spring onion to make a quick salsa.
- Poach the eggs by filling a saucepan full of boiling water from the kettle. Bring to a light simmer over a medium heat and season with salt.
- Crack each egg into a cup one at a time. Swirl the water gently with a spoon in a circular direction and carefully pour the egg into the water. Cook for 3 (soft) - 5 minutes (hard). Remove with a slotted spoon and place on kitchen paper to drain.
- Place the sausage meat in your bowl and top with your poached egg, avocado, sour cream, chopped coriander and sriracha sauce for attitude and optional keto tortilla chips.
- Best when served fresh, but can be stored in the fridge for 1 day.

Nutrition Info

Net carbs: 7.9 grams
Protein: 32.5 grams
Fat: 60 grams
Calories: 726 kcal

Anti Keto Flu Nourish Bowl

Most people experience keto flu at the beginning of their low carb journey. Caused by the change in your body due to starving it of carbohydrates, the keto flu feels like exactly that; the flu.

Prep/Cook Time: 20 minutes
Servings: 4

Ingredients

- 125g lupin flakes (4.4oz)
- 1 cup chicken broth or bone broth (240ml/8fl oz)
- 2 ½ cups chopped dark-leaf kale or spinach (125g/4.4oz)
- 1 ½ white mushrooms, sliced (105g/3.7oz)
- 1 can wild caught pink salmon, drained (150g/5.3oz)
- 1 tbsp ghee or virgin coconut oil (15ml)
- ¼ cup butter or ghee (60g/2.1oz)
- 1 clove garlic, minced
- ½ tsp sea salt, or to taste
- 1 large avocado, sliced (200g/7.1oz)
- 4 heaped tbsp hulled hemp seeds (60g/2.1oz)
- 2 tbsp extra virgin olive oil (30ml)
- Optional: chile flakes, to taste

Instructions

- Prepare all the ingredients. Clean and slice the mushrooms. Anti Keto Flu Nourish Bowl
- Place the lupin flakes into a microwaveable safe bowl and pour the chicken broth over. Stir through and sit aside for 15 minutes.
- Meanwhile, de-stem the kale and chop into small pieces. Finely mince the garlic.

- Heat half of the ghee in a frying pan over high heat and sauté the kale, along with the garlic, until softened but still bright green. If you're using spinach, it will only take about 30 seconds to wilt.
- Remove from pan and then cook mushrooms in the rest of the ghee in the pan. I like my mushrooms crispy on the outside and soft in the center, so I cook them well. Cook yours to your preferred doneness.
- Drain salmon and check through for bones.
- Once the lupin flakes have sat for 15 minutes, place them in the microwave for two minutes. Remove from the microwave and place pats of butter in to melt. Fluff up with a fork before serving. Anti Keto Flu Nourish Bowl
- Quarter your avocado and cut into slices.
- Gather your ingredients and arrange them in your bowl in the way you like (recipe makes 4 bowls). Sprinkle with salt and dress with a good sprinkle of hemp seeds. Optionally, you can add a sprinkle of chili flakes for extra heat or a squeeze of lemon juice, if you would like some added zing.
- Store in the refrigerator, without the avocado, covered for three days.

Nutrition Info

Net carbs: 3.9 grams
Protein: 31.9 grams
Fat: 42.8 grams
Calories: 558 kcal

Keto Portobello Mushroom Mini Pizzas

This low-carb recipe is also a great way to add in a ton of vegetables to your diet while keeping your carb intake low. Serve with a big bowl of green salad dressed in olive oil or homemade mayo and it's a great option if you practice intermittent fasting and need a high-energy, quick and easy meal to break your fast.

Prep/Cook Time: 20-25 minutes
Servings: 2

Ingredients

- 2 large portobello caps, stems removed (170g/ 6oz)
- ½ cup pesto (125g/4.4oz) -you can make your own pesto
- 10 black kalamata olives (30g/1.1oz)
- 1 tbsp canned peppers (10g/0.4oz)
- 1 tbsp capers (9g/0.3oz)
- 1 cup shredded Italian blend cheese (115g/4oz)
- Optional: pinch of crushed red pepper and basil for garnish

Instructions

- Preheat oven to 190 °C/ 375 °F (conventional), or 170 °C/ 340 °F (fan assisted) and place the mushrooms on a baking sheet. Divide the pesto between the mushrooms. (You can reserve the portobello stems and add them on top of your breakfast omelet.)
- Tip for the perfect portobellos: Baked mushrooms can be watery. To reduce the moisture, brush the portobellos with a small amount of ghee or olive oil and bake without the topping for 10-12 minutes. Add the topping and broil on high for another 2-3 minutes. Keto Portobello Mushroom Mini Pizzas

- Fill the centers with the cheese then top with your desired toppings.
- Bake for 10-15 minutes, just until the cheese is bubbly and the mushrooms are starting to soften.
- Serve immediately, optionally sprinkled with red pepper flakes, or refrigerate for up to a day and reheat before serving.

Note:

Apart from olives, pickled peppers and capers, you can top these mini pizzas with chopped sun-dried tomatoes, green olives, chopped pepperoni or bacon. Instead of pesto, you can use our homemade marinara sauce.

Nutrition Info

Net carbs: 6.8 grams
Protein: 18.6 grams
Fat: 60 grams
Calories: 646 kcal

Sugar-Free Lemon Granita

Prep/Cook Time: 3-4 hours
Servings: 8

Ingredients

- 2 cups fresh lemon juice, about 8 lemons (480ml/16 floz)
- zest from 1-2 organic lemons
- 3 cups filtered water (720ml/24fl oz)
- few sprigs of fresh thyme or mint
- ½ cup powdered Erythritol or Swerve (80g/2.8oz)
- pinch of sea salt
- Optional: few drops of stevia or more Erythritol to taste
- Optional: serve each glass with a shot of vodka or white rum

Instructions

- Zest 1 to 2 lemons and then juice all of them. Sugar-Free Lemon Granita
- Place the lemon juice, water, lemon zest, thyme leaves (or few mint leaves), Erythritol and salt into a blender. Process until smooth, for 15-20 seconds. Sugar-Free Lemon Granita
- Pour through a fine mesh sieve into a 1 ½ - 2 L container or baking dish that can fit into your freezer. Sugar-Free Lemon Granita
- Discard the pulp. Straining is required as the pulp may make the granita bitter. Sugar-Free Lemon Granita
- Freeze until the mixture becomes icy on the edges, about 30 minutes. Using a fork, scrape and mash the icy edges and combine with the unfrozen juices. Place back in the freezer and repeat up to 4 times, until the mixture is flaky - the granita is ready. Sugar-Free Lemon Granita

- To make the granita very smooth, scrape more with a fork, or place in a food processor and pulse until it resembles smooth snow. Sugar-Free Lemon Granita
- To serve, place the granita into serving glasses. Store any leftover granita in the freezer for up to 6 months. I like to keep mine in single-serving freezer bags. Sugar-Free Lemon Granita
- The granita can be served just like ice-cream, with a spoon, or frozen drink, with a straw. Optionally, add a shot of vodka or white rum. Sugar-Free Lemon Granita

Nutrition Info

Net carbs: 4.6 grams
Protein: 0.2 grams
Fat: 0.1 grams
Calories: 16 kcal

CONCLUSION

Intermittent fasting varies, but it is generally recommended for about one day every week. During this day, a person may have a liquid, nutrient-filled smoothie or other low-calorie option. As the body adjusts to an intermittent fasting regime, this usually is not necessary. Intermittent fasting helps to decrease fat stores naturally in the body, by switching the metabolism to break down fat instead of sugar or muscle. It has been used by many people effectively and is an easy way to make a beneficial change. For anyone who struggles with stubborn fat and is tired of traditional dieting, intermittent fasting offers an easy and effective option for fat loss and a healthier lifestyle.

Made in the USA
San Bernardino, CA
13 September 2019